Workout Your Way to Less Hunger

*How One Simple Exercise Routine
Can Help Control Cravings with
Extra Benefits for Women*

Tessy White

Table of Content

Introduction

Physical activity might not be the first thing that comes to mind when you want to control your hunger. More recent research, however, shows an interesting link between exercise and controlling your hunger, especially for women. Through a practical and scientifically sound method, this guide delves into the strong link between certain workouts and fewer cravings. It gives women the power to make healthier choices and enjoy the rewards of exercise beyond just fitness by helping them find a balance with food.

Handling hunger can be hard, especially for women. Differences in women's hunger habits are caused by biological factors like changes in hormones and body composition. Changes in hormones during the menstrual cycle, for example, can make cravings feel difficult or uncertain. However, the right exercise routine can play a key role in stabilizing these messages. Women can feel full and energized for longer after doing certain types of workouts because they lower amounts of hormones that make you hungry.

To what extent does this book specifically assist women? A customized method is needed first, since women's bodies have different needs and react differently to exercise than men's. What works for men to reduce hunger may not give the same results for women, and understanding these differences is important for making lasting changes. This guide is designed with these unique factors in mind, giving an easy-to-follow routine that aligns with women's physiology.

Developing this routine required looking closely at studies and expert insights into hunger-related hormones, such as ghrelin and leptin, and watching how they react to different exercises. The key focus became clear: it's not about working out harder or for longer; it's about picking the right combination of exercises. The program suggested here stresses strength training combined with low- to moderate-intensity cardio, a pairing that has been shown to promote fullness while preserving energy. This combination affects hunger hormones in a way that naturally helps control appetite without extreme dieting or restrictive habits.

By following this guide, women can experience a new relationship with exercise, one that isn't just about calories burned but is instead focused on long-term hunger control and general well-being. With a simple, research-based routine, the program tries to fit into any schedule while offering a manageable way to help women feel full and satisfied longer. This isn't just about temporary fixes or fad routines; it's about building a sustainable approach to exercise that truly makes a difference in daily life.

Chapter 1

The Science Behind Exercise and Hunger

Exercise does more than tone muscles or improve stamina; it also plays a fascinating part in managing hunger. At the center of this process are the hormones that regulate appetite, mainly ghrelin and leptin. Ghrelin, often called the "hunger hormone," signals our brain when it's time to eat, while leptin, the "satiety hormone," tells us when we're full. Physical exercise influences these hormones in a way that can help reduce cravings and extend feelings of fullness, making it easier to maintain a balanced eating pattern.

Physical activity, especially aerobic and strength training exercises, can reduce ghrelin levels in the short term, lowering the feeling of hunger right after a workout. Meanwhile, it boosts the body's sensitivity to leptin, which means that fullness cues become more effective over time. This normal adjustment makes it easier to avoid unnecessary snacking and overeating. The consistency of exercise, rather than its intensity, is key here; the more we engage in regular movement, the more responsive our bodies become to leptin, causing a steady cycle of feeling full and satisfied without additional calories.

For women, exercise offers unique hormonal benefits that go beyond hunger regulation. Due to fluctuations in estrogen and progesterone levels throughout the menstrual cycle, women often experience shifts in appetite, energy, and even food choices. Exercise can be particularly helpful in balancing these changes. For instance, studies have shown that aerobic activities such as brisk walking or light running can help lower estrogen levels post-exercise, which can stabilize mood and hunger. Furthermore, strength training has been shown to positively affect metabolic rate and blood sugar levels, helping women keep energy and reduce cravings for sugary or high-carb foods.

In recent years, researchers have been especially interested in understanding how specific workouts affect hunger regulation. One key study found that women who participated in a moderate exercise routine experienced a measurable reduction in ghrelin levels compared to those who did not exercise. This result shows that exercise directly impacts hunger control, especially with routines that combine cardio and strength. Another study focusing on long-term exercise habits found that women who regularly exercised had lower ghrelin levels and higher leptin sensitivity, suggesting that exercise offers enduring appetite control benefits.

These results emphasize that, for women, a consistent, balanced exercise routine can make all the difference in appetite control. Through knowing how physical activity impacts hunger hormones, women can leverage exercise as a natural, sustainable way to manage cravings, achieve a balanced diet, and enjoy overall wellness. This information supports a shift from exercising purely for fitness to working out with the added intention of managing hunger and enhancing quality of life.

Chapter 2

Crafting Your Hunger-Reducing Workout Routine

Creating a hunger-reducing workout plan is all about balance and personalization. To make a workout plan that truly helps manage cravings, it's important to focus on exercises that regulate hunger hormones, improve energy, and enhance general well-being. This routine doesn't require extreme effort or endless hours in the gym; instead, it's built around consistent, manageable activities that fit easily into any lifestyle. Let's explore the essential components of this workout plan, including the optimal frequency, length, and intensity, as well as tips for tailoring the routine to suit various fitness levels.

At its core, the hunger-reducing workout practice is a mix of strength training, aerobic exercise, and gentle stretching. Strength training, like lifting weights or using resistance bands, is key to building lean muscle, which in turn helps control appetite by boosting metabolism and stabilizing blood sugar levels. This stability helps avoid cravings, especially for quick-energy foods like sweets or refined carbs. Aerobic exercises, such as walking, cycling, or low-impact dance workouts, are equally important; they have been shown to lower ghrelin levels and improve leptin sensitivity, giving the body a natural hunger-regulating effect. Finally, stretching or yoga rounds out the process, promoting relaxation and lowering cortisol, which can reduce stress-related cravings.

To achieve the best results, finding the right frequency, duration, and intensity is important. Ideally, the workout plan includes four to five days of exercise each week. Three days can focus on moderate aerobic exercise, with each session lasting around 30 to 45 minutes. Two days can be saved for strength training, with 20 to 30 minutes dedicated to exercises targeting major muscle groups, such as the legs, back, and core. These sessions should be moderate in intensity; workouts don't need to be strenuous to have good effects on hunger control. In fact, overly intense sessions can sometimes raise cortisol, which may lead to cravings. A steady, moderate approach promotes consistency, making it easier to stick with the routine in the long run.

Customization is the key to making this plan successful and sustainable, especially for different fitness levels. For beginners, start slow by focusing on low-impact aerobic activities like brisk walks, and use lighter weights for strength training. Gradually increase the length and intensity as your stamina improves. Intermediate and advanced people can aim for more varied cardio options, like interval training, which alternates between high- and low-intensity exercises to maximize calorie burn and appetite control. For strength training, incorporating more challenging weights or resistance bands can further improve muscle tone and metabolic stability.

This hunger-reducing workout routine offers flexibility and can be changed based on personal preferences, schedules, and goals. By combining these essential components—strength, aerobic exercise, and stretching—at an appropriate frequency, length, and intensity, the routine creates a balanced approach to hunger management. It's a sustainable way to not only feel stronger and more energized but also keep better control over cravings and feel more in tune with hunger cues.

Chapter 3

Step-by-Step Hunger-Reducing Exercises

A well-designed hunger-reducing workout starts with mindful movement and builds through exercises that are proven to help curb cravings and support overall wellness. Each step has a specific purpose: from warming up to activating your metabolism, to performing targeted exercises that control hunger hormones, to ending with cool-down stretches that help your body recover and relax. Here's a step-by-step guide to each part of this hunger-reducing workout practice.

Warm-Up Essentials to Activate Metabolism

Before diving into the main exercises, start with a 5- to 10-minute warm-up to slowly increase your heart rate and activate your metabolism. Warm-up moves should focus on active (moving) stretches that prepare your muscles for the workout ahead. Begin with light jogging in place or brisk walking, followed by moves like arm circles, leg swings, and high knees. These dynamic moves not only warm up your muscles but also stimulate blood flow, ensuring that your body is ready to maximize energy and hunger-regulating benefits during the workout.

Primary Exercises for Appetite Control

Once warmed up, move into exercises meant to specifically help with appetite control. These are usually moderate-intensity moves that balance cardio with strength-building elements. Here are some useful options:

Bodyweight Squats: Stand with your feet hip-width apart, bend at the knees and drop into a squat, then rise back up. This full-body move works the largest muscle groups and boosts metabolism, supporting better hunger control.

Plank: Position yourself face-down, elbows beneath shoulders, legs tucked under, and lift your body into a straight line. Hold for 20–30 seconds. This core exercise stabilizes blood sugar levels, which helps avoid energy dips that can lead to cravings.

Mountain Climbers: Start in a plank pose and bring one knee toward your chest, then quickly alternate legs. This move combines cardio and core strengthening, successfully reducing ghrelin levels that signal hunger.

Walking Lunges: Take a step forward and lower into a lunge, alternating knees as you move. Lunges target large muscles, improving calorie burn and satiety levels post-workout.

Strength Training Basics

Strength training is important for building lean muscle, which not only shapes the body but also stabilizes blood sugar levels, reducing the risk of cravings. Strength moves should be done at least twice a week and focus on compound movements that target multiple muscles at once.

Dumbbell Deadlifts: With feet hip-width apart, hold dumbbells in front of your legs. Bend at the hips, dropping the dumbbells along your legs, then return to standing. This move works the back, hamstrings, and glutes—muscle groups that rev up metabolism and support appetite control.

Push-Ups: A classic but useful strength move. If a full push-up is too difficult, modify by doing them on your knees. Push-ups engage the chest, shoulders, and triceps, adding to a balanced body and helping reduce ghrelin levels.

Shoulder Press: Using light dumbbells, hold weights at shoulder height, and press them upward, then lower back down. This upper-body move stabilizes blood sugar and keeps hunger hormones in check, especially post-workout.

Cardio Routines for Maximum Impact

Cardio plays a key role in this workout plan by burning calories and supporting leptin sensitivity, which helps the body better recognize when it's full. The key is modest intensity—enough to break a sweat without pushing yourself to exhaustion.

Brisk Walking or Light Jogging: A 20–30 minute walk or light jog is useful and accessible. Walking or jogging at a moderate pace has been shown to reduce ghrelin, making you feel less hungry afterward.

Interval Training: For those with a bit more energy, try intervals. Alternate between 1 minute of moderate walking and 1 minute of fast-paced running. Repeat for 20 minutes. Interval training maximizes calorie burn and appetite regulation, perfect for those with limited time.

Cycling: Cycling, either outdoors or on a stationary bike, for 20–30 minutes at a moderate speed can also regulate hunger hormones. Cycling targets big muscle groups, increasing energy expenditure and lowering post-workout cravings.

Cool-Down and Stretching for Recovery

Cooling down helps reduce muscle soreness and prevents injury while telling the body that the workout is complete. More importantly, it calms cortisol levels, which, when high, can cause cravings for sugary or high-calorie foods.

Forward Fold: Stand tall, then slowly fold forward, reaching toward your toes. This stretch relaxes the hamstrings and lower back, promoting relaxation and reducing stress-related cravings.

Seated Twist: Sit with your legs extended, cross one leg over the other, and slowly twist toward the bent knee. This stretch releases tension in the back and promotes a calm mind.

Child's Pose: Kneel on the floor, sit back on your heels, and stretch your arms forward, bringing your chest toward the floor. This relaxed position stretches the back, shoulders, and hips, while calming the nervous system.

Deep Breathing: Finish with a few minutes of deep breathing. Take a relaxed seat, close your eyes, and breathe deeply in and out. This final step lowers cortisol and leaves you feeling mentally and physically balanced.

By following this structured routine—warming up, performing main hunger-regulating exercises, focusing on strength and cardio, and finishing with a cool-down—you create a sustainable workout that supports hunger control. Over time, this habit can help you achieve a better balance between exercise and appetite, reducing cravings naturally and supporting a healthy lifestyle.

Chapter 4

Enhancing Hunger Control with Lifestyle Adjustments

Exercise plays a huge role in managing hunger, but it's only one piece of the picture. Lifestyle factors like mindfulness, hydration, and quality sleep work hand-in-hand with physical exercise to help you feel more satisfied and maintain control over cravings. By adjusting daily habits around exercise, you can set yourself up for long-term success in controlling hunger and sustaining energy levels. Let's study how to improve hunger control through mindfulness, hydration, and sleep.

Integrating Mindfulness into Workouts

Mindfulness, or the practice of being fully present in the moment, can have a changing effect on workouts and appetite control. When we approach exercise with intention and awareness, we're less likely to overdo it, which helps avoid the spike in hunger that often follows overly intense sessions. Practicing mindfulness during workouts also helps you stay in tune with your body's needs, making it easier to notice natural hunger and satiety cues.

To add mindfulness, try focusing on your breathing during exercise. Notice each inhale and exhale as you move through each set or exercise. If running or walking, pay attention to how your feet hit the ground or how your muscles feel as they work. You can also try a body scan at the end of your session—mentally check in with each part of your body to notice any areas of stress or relaxation. This mental focus not only improves your workout experience but also builds a stronger connection between exercise and well-being, making you less prone to mindless snacking afterward.

Hydration Tips for Reduced Cravings

Staying hydrated is one of the easiest yet most effective strategies for hunger control. Our brains can sometimes mix thirst with hunger, leading to unnecessary snacking or cravings, especially for salty or sugary foods. Drinking enough water helps keep this confusion at bay, making it easier to distinguish real hunger from a thirst signal.

To keep optimal hydration, aim to drink water consistently throughout the day instead of trying to "catch up" all at once. Start your day with a glass of water, as this can help wake up your body and prevent morning cravings. During workouts, sip water regularly to replace fluids lost through sweat, and try to keep a water bottle nearby to make it handy. Infusing water with lemon, cucumber, or mint can make it more enjoyable if you're not usually drawn to plain water. Additionally, consider hydrating with electrolytes if you're doing longer or high-intensity workouts, as they can help restore important minerals without adding unnecessary sugars that might spark cravings.

How Sleep Influences Appetite and Performance

A good night's sleep is one of the most underrated tools for hunger control and workout success. Quality sleep helps the body to regulate the hormones ghrelin and leptin effectively—two primary hormones involved in appetite. When we're sleep-deprived, ghrelin (the hunger hormone) tends to rise, while leptin (the satiety hormone) decreases, resulting in increased cravings and trouble feeling full. Research shows that people who get inadequate sleep often experience heightened cravings for high-calorie foods, which can make it challenging to keep balanced eating habits.

To support hunger control, try for seven to nine hours of restful sleep each night. Prioritize a regular sleep routine, even on weekends, to help regulate your body's internal clock. Creating a calming bedtime practice can improve sleep quality, as can reducing screen time and avoiding heavy meals or caffeine close to bedtime. Good sleep not only helps with managing appetite but also improves exercise performance by improving focus, energy levels, and muscle recovery, making it easier to stick to your workout routine and manage hunger over the long term.

By enhancing hunger control through mindfulness, hydration, and quality sleep, you build a strong foundation for managing cravings and improving well-being. These lifestyle changes complement the hunger-reducing workout routine, ensuring that your approach to appetite control is well-rounded and sustainable. With a mindful attitude, steady hydration, and restorative sleep, you'll find it easier to connect with your body's true needs, making it simpler to enjoy a balanced approach to fitness, hunger, and health.

Chapter 5

Eating to Support Your Workout Goals

To effectively control hunger and support your workout goals, nutrition plays a pivotal role. The right foods not only provide the energy needed for physical exercise but also help control appetite and enhance recovery. By choosing nutrient-dense options, timing your meals carefully, and following structured meal plans, you can create a sustainable eating approach that complements your hunger-reducing workout routine. Let's dive into a nutrition guide meant to support your fitness objectives and control cravings.

Foods That Naturally Suppress Appetite

Incorporating specific foods into your diet can help keep hunger at bay while still providing important nutrients for your body. Here are some food groups to consider:

High-Fiber Foods: Foods rich in fiber take longer to digest, which helps keep you feeling fuller for longer. Consider incorporating whole grains (like oats and quinoa), legumes (such as beans and lentils), and plenty of fruits and veggies (like apples, berries, broccoli, and carrots) into your meals.

Lean Proteins: Protein is known to increase satiety and reduce hunger. Include sources like chicken, turkey, fish, eggs, Greek yogurt, and plant-based proteins such as tofu or tempeh in your diet. These foods help balance blood sugar levels and keep muscle mass, which is crucial for effective workouts.

Healthy Fats: Contrary to popular opinion, healthy fats can help control appetite by promoting feelings of fullness. Foods such as avocados, nuts, seeds, and olive oil are great picks. They provide essential fatty acids that support general health while keeping hunger in check.

Hydrating Foods: Foods with high water content, like cucumbers, tomatoes, and watermelon, can help you stay hydrated and feel full without adding many calories.

Incorporating these into your meals can help in managing cravings effectively.

Timing Meals with Workouts for Best Results

Meal timing can significantly impact your workout ability and appetite control. Here are some tips to follow:

Pre-Workout Nutrition: Consuming a balanced meal or snack about 1 to 3 hours before your workout can provide the energy needed for best performance. Aim for a mix of carbohydrates and protein—think oatmeal topped with fruit and a dollop of yogurt or a smoothie with spinach, banana, and protein powder.

Post-Workout repair: After exercising, it's crucial to replenish your body's energy stores and support muscle repair. Ideally, eat a meal or snack within 30 to 60 minutes post-workout. This should include protein for muscle repair and carbohydrates to recover glycogen levels. A protein shake with a banana or a chicken salad with quinoa and mixed vegetables are great options.

Regular Meal Patterns: Eating smaller, balanced meals throughout the day can help stabilize blood sugar levels and avoid excessive hunger. Try to include a mix of protein, healthy fats, and complex carbohydrates in each meal to support sustained energy and satiety.

Sample Meal Plans for Women Focused on Craving Control

Here's a simple meal plan designed to support workout goals while helping control cravings:

Meal Plan 1:

Breakfast: Greek yogurt with mixed berries and a sprinkle of chia seeds.

Mid-Morning Snack: A small handful of peanuts and an apple.

Lunch: Quinoa salad with beans, diced cucumbers, cherry tomatoes, and a drizzle of olive oil.

Afternoon Snack: Carrot sticks with hummus.

Dinner: Grilled salmon with steamed broccoli and sweet potato.

Evening Snack: A small bowl of air-popped popcorn.

Meal Plan 2:

Breakfast: Scrambled eggs with spinach and whole-grain toast.

Mid-Morning Snack: A shake made with banana, spinach, and protein powder.

Lunch: Turkey wrap with whole-grain bread, lettuce, tomatoes, and avocado.

Afternoon Snack: Cottage cheese with pineapple chunks.

Dinner: Stir-fried tofu with mixed veggies served over brown rice.

Evening Snack: Sliced cucumber with a dash of salt and pepper.

Meal Plan 3:

Breakfast: Overnight oats made with rolled oats, almond milk, and topped with sliced bananas.

Mid-Morning Snack: A boiled egg and a few small tomatoes.

Lunch: Lentil soup with a side of mixed veggies drizzled with balsamic vinaigrette.

Afternoon Snack: Sliced bell peppers with guacamole.

Dinner: Baked chicken breast with vegetables and quinoa.

Evening Snack: A small piece of dark chocolate and a cup of herbal tea.

By incorporating these hunger-suppressing foods, timing your meals effectively, and following these sample meal plans, you can create a supportive nutrition strategy that improves your workout goals and helps manage cravings. Remember that consistency is key; making these habits part of your daily routine can lead to long-term success in both exercise and appetite control.

Chapter 6

Hormones, Hunger, and Women's Health

Hormones play a significant role in regulating hunger, influencing energy levels, and impacting overall health, especially for women. Understanding the interplay between hormones like estrogen, ghrelin, and leptin can provide useful insights into managing hunger and optimizing workout routines. Additionally, recognizing how menstrual cycles affect these hormones helps women to adapt their exercise and nutrition strategies accordingly. Here's a deeper look into hormones, hunger, and women's health.

Understanding Estrogen, Ghrelin, and Leptin

Estrogen, ghrelin, and leptin are crucial hormones that affect hunger and energy regulation.

Estrogen: This main female sex hormone is not only important for reproductive health but also plays a role in appetite regulation. Higher levels of estrogen are often linked with reduced appetite, while lower levels can lead to increased hunger. Estrogen also affects the distribution of body fat, which can further influence how the body reacts to hunger signals.

Ghrelin: Known as the "hunger hormone," ghrelin is produced in the stomach and tells the brain when it's time to eat. Levels of ghrelin usually rise before meals and decrease after eating. Research shows that women may experience higher ghrelin levels during certain stages of their menstrual cycles, leading to increased hunger and cravings.

Leptin: Often referred to as the "satiety hormone," leptin is produced by fat cells and tells the brain to stop eating. It helps control energy balance by inhibiting hunger. Leptin levels can be affected by body fat, sleep quality, and physical activity. Women with higher body fat may have higher leptin levels, but they may also become resistant to its effects, leading to problems in appetite control.

How Menstrual Cycles Influence Hunger and Workout Efficiency

The menstrual cycle consists of different phases, each characterized by varying hormone levels, which can greatly affect hunger and exercise ability.

Follicular Phase: During this phase, estrogen levels rise, usually leading to reduced appetite and increased energy levels. This is often considered an ideal time for women to engage in high-intensity workouts, as energy levels are usually higher and workouts may feel more manageable.

Ovulation: Around ovulation, estrogen peaks, which can lead to a brief rise in energy and possibly higher libido. Many women may experience a natural boost in workout ability during this time. Appetite tends to stay stable, allowing for more effective exercise sessions.

Luteal Phase: After ovulation, estrogen levels drop while progesterone rises. This time can bring about increased hunger and cravings, often for carbohydrate-rich foods. As energy levels may dip, women might find themselves feeling more fatigued, which can impact workout intensity and drive. Adjusting the workout routine to include more moderate-intensity exercises or focusing on lighter strength training can be helpful during this time.

Adapting the Routine to Support Hormonal Balance

To optimize workouts and manage hunger effectively, it's essential to change routines in line with hormonal fluctuations throughout the menstrual cycle. Here are some methods to consider:

Tailoring Workouts: Listen to your body and change the intensity of your workouts based on where you are in your cycle. During the follicular phase and ovulation, aim for higher-intensity workouts such as interval training or strength classes. In the luteal phase, consider adding more low-impact exercises like yoga, walking, or light resistance training, which can help reduce fatigue and promote relaxation.

Nutrient Adjustments: Pay attention to your body's nutrient needs throughout the cycle. In the luteal phase, focus on incorporating complex carbohydrates, healthy fats, and protein to help handle increased cravings and keep energy levels. Foods like whole grains, nuts, seeds, and legumes can provide prolonged energy while supporting hormonal balance.

Mindfulness Practices: Incorporating mindfulness practices such as meditation or gentle stretching can improve mental well-being and help manage cravings during the luteal phase. Mindfulness can also improve attention and motivation during workouts, making them more enjoyable.

Adequate Sleep and Recovery: Prioritize sleep and recovery, especially during the luteal phase when tiredness can set in. Aim for 7-9 hours of quality sleep each night to support hormonal regulation and general health. Rest days or active recovery days should be planned carefully to align with your body's needs.

By understanding the relationships between hormones, hunger, and women's health, you can make informed choices that support your fitness goals and improve well-being. Adapting workout routines and nutrition strategies based on hormonal changes will not only help manage cravings but also improve exercise efficiency, leading to a healthier and more balanced lifestyle.

Chapter 7

Managing Challenges and Staying Motivated

Staying motivated and overcoming obstacles are key components of any fitness journey, especially when it comes to managing hunger and maintaining workout routines. Everyone meets obstacles like fatigue, workout plateaus, and fluctuations in appetite, but how you react to these challenges can make all the difference. Let's explore effective strategies for overcoming common barriers, keeping consistency with appetite goals, and creating a supportive environment that fosters success.

Fatigue and workout plateaus can be frustrating, but they are often a natural part of the fitness path. Here are some tips for beating these hurdles:

Listen to Your Body: If fatigue strikes, it's important to listen to your body. Consider adding rest days or active recovery days, such as gentle yoga or leisurely walks. Rest is crucial for muscle recovery and can help avoid burnout, allowing you to return to your workouts feeling refreshed and re-energized.

Change Your Routine: If you find yourself hitting a halt, it might be time to switch things up. This can mean trying new exercises, altering the intensity of your workouts, or varying your schedule to include different types of physical activities. Variety not only helps keep workouts interesting but also challenges your body in new ways, supporting progress.

Set Realistic Goals: Instead of looking for drastic changes, focus on small, achievable goals. Whether it's increasing your weights, adding an extra set to your workout, or incorporating a new type of exercise, celebrating small victories can boost your motivation and keep you involved.

Stay Hydrated and Nourished: Fatigue can often stem from inadequate hydration or nutrients. Make sure to drink plenty of water throughout the day and fuel your body with nutrient-dense foods that provide steady energy. Eating balanced meals rich in protein, healthy fats, and carbohydrates will help keep you motivated during workouts.

Staying Consistent with Appetite Goals

Consistency is key when it comes to managing appetite and meeting your fitness goals. Here are some methods to help you stay on track:

Establish a schedule: Create a consistent daily schedule for meals, snacks, and workouts. This can help regulate your body's hunger signals and make it easier to avoid unhealthy cravings. Try to eat at similar times each day and incorporate regular workout sessions into your routine.

Mindful Eating: Practice mindful eating by paying attention to your hunger cues and eating slowly. This approach allows you to enjoy your food, recognize when you're full, and avoid overeating. Keeping a food journal can also help track your meals, monitor hunger levels, and spot patterns in cravings.

Accountability: Share your goals with friends or family members who can help hold you accountable. Whether it's through check-ins, sharing meal plans, or working out together, having a support system can reinforce your commitment to controlling appetite and staying consistent with your routine.

Reward Yourself: Celebrate your progress, no matter how small. Set up a reward system for achieving specific milestones linked to appetite control or fitness achievements. Whether it's treating yourself to a massage, a new workout outfit, or a fun outing, acknowledging your hard work can keep you inspired.

Building a Supportive Environment for Success

Creating a supportive setting is crucial for sustaining motivation and overcoming obstacles. Here are some ways to build an inspiring atmosphere:

Surround Yourself with Positivity: Engage with supportive friends, family members, or exercise groups who share similar goals. A positive support network can motivate you to stay committed and make the journey more enjoyable.

Remove Temptations: If certain foods trigger cravings or unhealthy eating habits, consider minimizing their presence in your home. Stock your kitchen with healthy options and make snacks that align with your appetite goals. This way, you'll be less likely to reach for unhealthy choices when hunger hits.

Create a Motivational Space: Designate a particular area in your home for workouts and meal prep. This place should be free from distractions and filled with items that inspire you, such as workout gear, motivational quotes, or visuals representing your goals.

Use Technology Wisely: Utilize exercise apps or wearable devices that track your workouts and nutrition. These tools can help you stay responsible and provide insights into your progress. Many apps also offer community features where you can meet with others on similar journeys, adding an extra layer of support.

By developing strategies to overcome fatigue and plateaus, staying consistent with appetite goals, and building a supportive environment, you can handle challenges more effectively and maintain motivation on your fitness journey. Remember, it's okay to face setbacks; what counts is how you respond and keep moving forward.

Conclusion

When it comes to managing hunger through exercise, many questions and myths can cause confusion. This part will address some of the most common questions people have about the relationship between hunger and exercise, debunk popular myths, and outline key dos and don'ts for effective hunger control.

Addressing Popular Myths Myth: Exercising Always Suppresses Hunger While many people find that exercise can reduce their appetite, the benefits can vary from person to person. Some may experience an increase in hunger after intense workouts, especially if they are engaged in long-duration or high-intensity exercises. It's important to listen to your body and understand that hunger responses can be affected by various factors, including the type of exercise, duration, and individual metabolism.

Myth: Skipping Meals Before Workouts Helps Burn More Fat Skipping meals before exercising may seem like a good way to boost fat burning, but it can lead to increased hunger later and diminished workout performance. Not fueling your body properly can result in fatigue, reduced intensity during workouts, and an increased chance of overeating after exercising. It's usually more effective to eat a balanced meal or snack before working out.

Myth: All Carbs Are Bad for Managing Hunger Carbohydrates often get a bad rap, but they play a crucial role in fueling workouts and controlling appetite. The key is to focus on eating complex carbohydrates, such as whole grains, fruits, and vegetables, which provide sustained energy and help keep you feeling full. Simple carbohydrates, on the other hand, can lead to rapid spikes and drops in blood sugar, resulting in greater hunger.

Myth: You Can Out-Exercise a Poor Diet While regular exercise is important for general health, it's not a substitute for a balanced diet. Exercise and nutrition work together to support appetite control, energy levels, and general well-being. Relying solely on exercise to offset bad dietary choices can lead to weight gain and other health issues over time.

Dos and Don'ts for Hunger Control Through Exercise

Do Listen to Your Body: Pay attention to your food cues and energy levels. If you're feeling hungry after a workout, allow yourself to refuel with a healthy snack or meal that includes a mix of protein, healthy fats, and complex carbs.

Do Incorporate a Variety of Exercises: Mix different types of workouts, such as strength training, cardio, and flexibility movements. This variety can help keep you focused and motivated while supporting appetite control.

Do Stay Hydrated: Dehydration can sometimes be mistaken for hunger. Make sure to drink plenty of water throughout the day, especially before, during, and after workouts, to stay hydrated and help control your appetite.

Do Practice Mindful Eating: Focus on your meals and snacks, enjoying each bite. Eating mindfully can help you notice your body's hunger signals and prevent overeating.

Do Set Realistic Goals: Aim for gradual changes in your exercise and nutrition routines. Setting achievable goals can help you stay motivated and keep a consistent approach to managing hunger.

Don't Skip Meals Regularly: Regularly skipping meals can lead to greater hunger and cravings later in the day, making it harder to stick to healthy eating habits.

Instead, aim for healthy meals and snacks throughout the day.

Don't Rely on Exercise Alone for Weight Loss: While exercise is an important component of a healthy lifestyle, it's not the only factor in weight management. Focus on a holistic approach that includes balanced nutrition and regular physical exercise.

Don't Ignore Post-Workout Nutrition: After exercising, it's important to refuel your body to aid recovery and avoid excessive hunger later. Make sure to consume a healthy meal or snack that includes protein and carbohydrates within an hour of finishing your workout.

Don't Fall for Quick-Fix Diets: Avoid fad diets that promise rapid weight loss without sustainable living changes. Instead, focus on long-term strategies that support healthy eating and regular exercise.

Don't Compare Yourself to Others: Everyone's body acts differently to exercise and hunger. Focus on your individual journey, and understand that progress may look different for everyone.

www.ingramcontent.com/pod-product-compliance
Lightning Source LLC
Chambersburg PA
CBHW061520250726
48657CB00005B/1983